STAYING

HEALTHY

KEEP FIT!

Miriam Moss

Wayland

STAYING HEALTHY

BE POSITIVE!
BODY CARE
EAT WELL!
KEEP FIT!

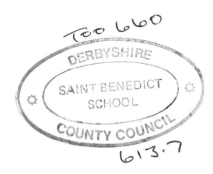

Series editor: Kathryn Smith
Series designer: Helen White

First published in 1992 by
Wayland (Publishers) Ltd
61 Western Road, Hove
East Sussex, BN3 1JD England

British Library Cataloguing in Publication Data

Moss, Miriam
Keep fit. – (Staying Healthy)
I. Title II. Series
613.7
ISBN 0 75 02 0368 4

Typeset by White Design.
Printed by Canale & C.S.p.A, in Turin.
Bound by A.G.M. in France.

CONTENTS

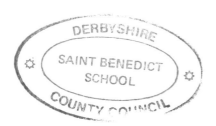

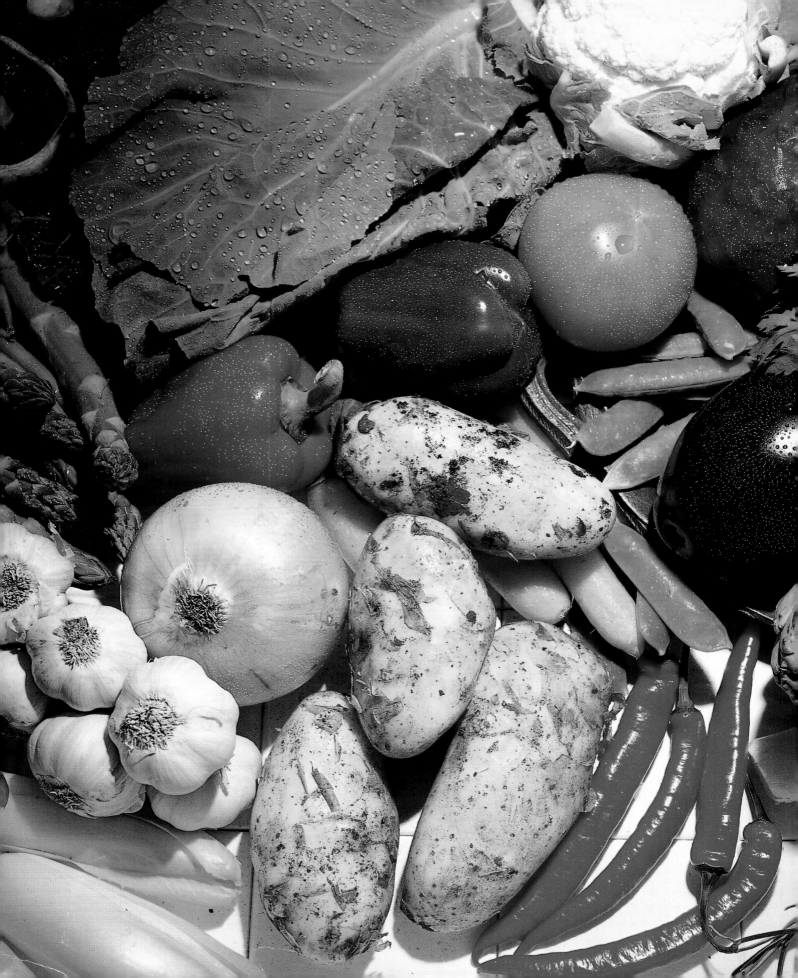

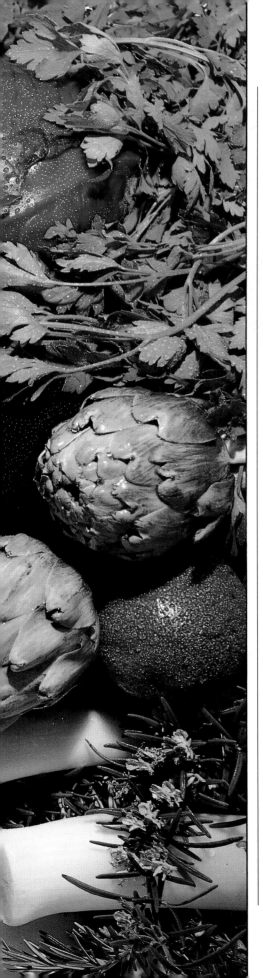

HEALTHY LIFESTYLES

How fit are you ?
Do you get out of breath when you run for a bus? Do you eat plenty of fresh fruit and vegetables or do you prefer a quick hamburger and chips? Are you active, taking regular exercise or do you always choose the lazy way of doing things?

You've probably heard people say: 'Exercise? No, I'm not the sporty type. It's too much like hard work, what I need is a rest. Anyway, I'd never be able to keep it up, I'm too busy.' Maybe you say it too, but being fit doesn't have to hurt and it doesn't have to take up much time either. Fitness means that you can do more for less effort - and that makes sense!

An easy lifestyle threatens your health because your body is not designed for inactivity. You need exercise to keep your body strong and flexible. Without regular exercise your muscles, including your heart, become less efficient. Strengthening your heart helps you to resist heart disease, colds, flu and other infections and it keeps your whole system healthy.

◀ **Fresh raw vegetables are packed with essential nutrients.**

▼ **How profitably do you think you spend your leisure time?**

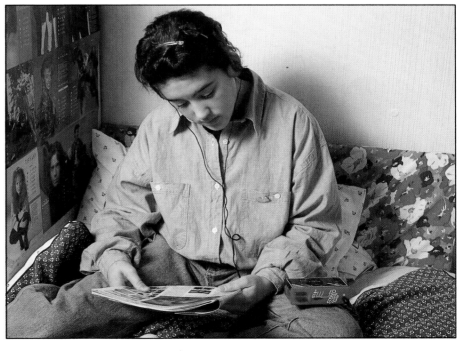

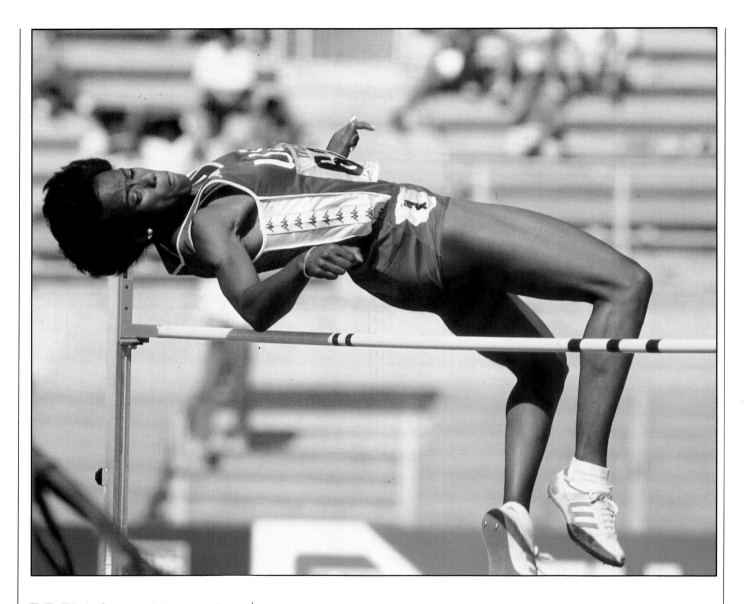

What is good health ?

Being healthy does not just mean that you are not ill. As well as being physically fit and well, you need to feel good about the way you are and about your lifestyle. Health is to do with the whole person: it is a combination of the body and mind functioning well.

Fitness is an important part of being healthy. Being fit can make you feel happier and more confident about yourself. You will have more energy too. Your level of fitness shows in how supple you are and how much strength and stamina you have. Regular exercise is the only way to become really fit - there are no short cuts.

The World Health Organization (WHO) defines health as:
'... complete economic, physical, mental and social well-being. But one of the best measures of health is how each individual accepts and adapts to their own limitations.'

▲ To maintain peak fitness, world class athletes like Jackie Joyner-Kersee have to be dedicated and determined.

▶ If you decide to improve your fitness level, do not be too ambitious at first. You can do simple exercises such as sit-ups in your bedroom, building up strength and stamina gradually.

Do you have a choice ?

You cannot always choose the conditions in which you live, how rich or poor you are, or the kind of lifestyle your family leads. Neither can you choose your body shape or other inherited characteristics like the colour of your eyes or your height. We are all born different. Some people are born with disabilities. However, people with disabilities can also enjoy certain sports and other forms of exercise to keep fit and healthy.

You can choose to take responsibility for your own body. If you pay attention to the health education available to you, you can choose a fulfilling lifestyle. With it you can learn how to avoid illness, making sure, for example, that you are protected against disease through immunization programmes. If you are well informed you can improve your diet and also avoid risking your health through drinking too much alcohol, smoking cigarettes or taking illegal drugs.

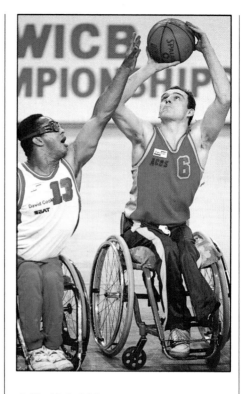

▲ Disabled athletes enjoy a wide range of sporting activities at all levels.

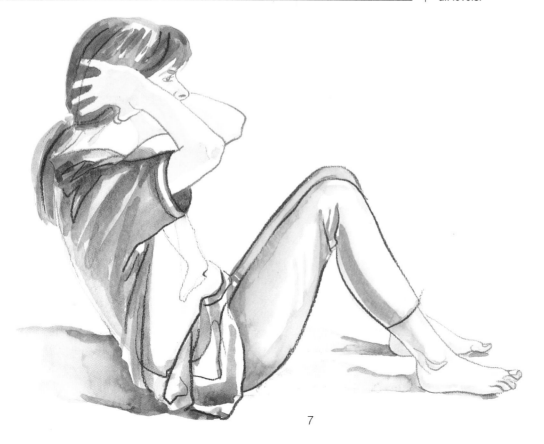

WHY EXERCISE ?

What's in it for me ?
The good news is that exercise is fun! The right combination of activities makes you happier, healthier, fitter and in better shape than ever before. You feel more energetic and it gets easier the more you do. Exercising is a great way of making new friends and enjoying your leisure time. It also helps you to relax, making you feel good in mind and body. It increases the rate at which you burn off calories, helping you to get slim and stay slim. It helps almost everything in your body work better, keeping you supple, strengthening your muscles, joints and bones, and improving your circulation.

What happens when you exercise ?
When you exercise you use your muscles to move your bones. To do this you need energy which you get through the food you eat.

◀ Team sports such as tennis enable you to stay fit and meet new friends.

▶ These young hurdlers burn up a huge number of calories to obtain the energy necessary to run at high speed.

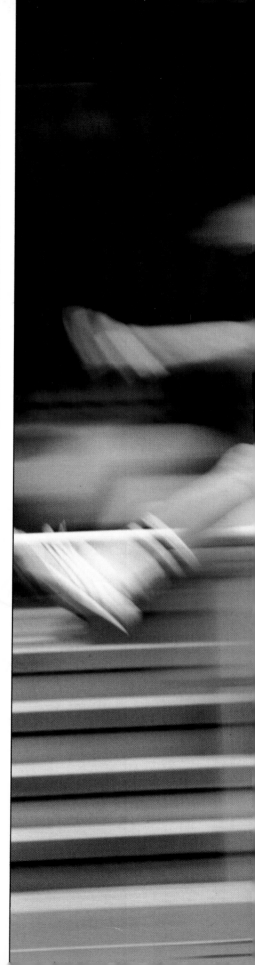

8

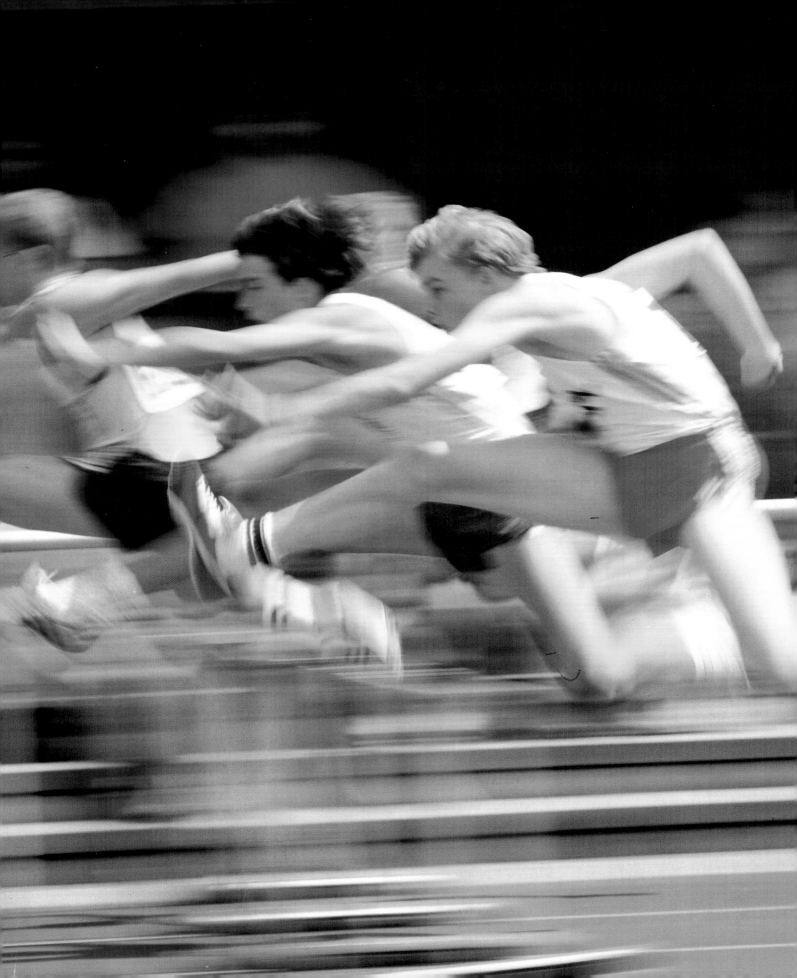

Look after your heart

Heart disease develops when harmful fatty substances build up inside the arteries carrying blood to the heart muscle. Exercise gets the blood moving rapidly through the arteries, stopping the deposits from building up so easily. Blood pressure is the force with which the heart muscle squirts blood through your arteries. Smoking, lack of exercise, being overweight or being subject to too much stress can make your arteries deteriorate. Then your blood pressure rises. This is because your heart has to pump harder to force the blood through the damaged blood vessels to carry the same amount of oxygen to your muscles. Regular exercise helps blood vessels open up and gives your heart an easier time.

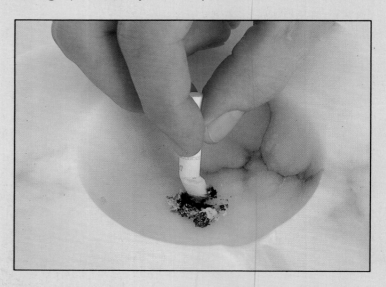

Oxygen is needed to release the energy. The oxygen in the air you breathe gets to your muscles via your lungs and blood system. When you exercise your muscles work harder and use up more oxygen. Exercise makes muscles more efficient at using oxygen to perform work. It strengthens your chest muscles and increases the amount of air your lungs can hold, as well as strengthening the heart muscles which pump blood around the body.

Aerobic exercise

Your heart, lungs and blood system together are called your aerobic system. Aerobic exercise strengthens your aerobic system and makes it function efficiently.

▲ Smoking is not only bad for your heart and lungs, but it makes your clothes, hair and breath smell stale.

▼ Linford Christie powers down the track. Running helps to make your heart and lungs work more efficiently.

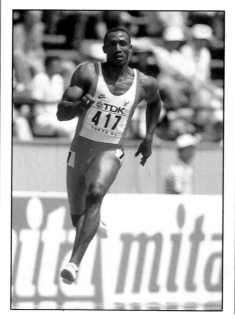

It is the kind of exercise which you can sustain for long periods at a steady pace – like jogging, skipping or cycling. You should aim to build at least three half-hour sessions into your weekly routine. The chart on page 11 shows how different aerobic exercises burn up calories.

Stored fat

The food that you eat gives you energy which helps you to grow and keeps your body working properly. Regular exercise uses up the energy that is produced from the food you eat. If you eat more food than you need and don't exercise then you may become overweight. Spare calories are stored in the form of fat. Being seriously overweight puts strain on your heart and joints, raises your blood pressure and increases your chances of being diabetic. There is no doubt that you look and feel better if you keep your body slim and toned-up and your weight at the proper level for your size.

Most teenagers have very fit bodies but many worry unnecessarily about their shape. This is often because of unreasonable pressure from the media for people's body shapes to conform to those set by fashion. The best way to stay healthy is to combine healthy eating with exercise and to be determined not to let your fitness deteriorate as you approach your twenties.

Burn it up

The speed at which you convert food into energy is called your metabolic rate. Different people have different metabolic rates. If you have a fast rate then you may be able to eat a lot

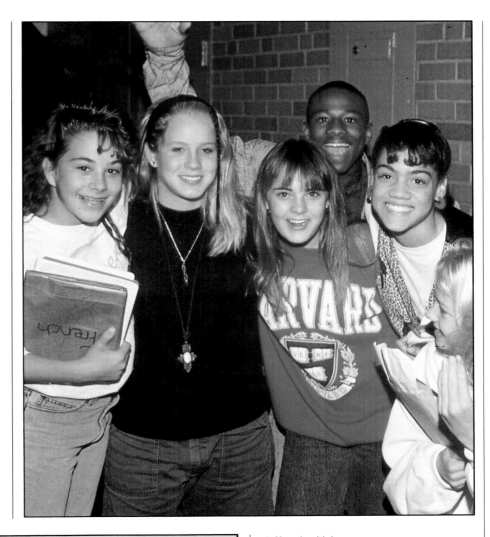

▲ Your health is precious. It makes sense to stay healthy by keeping fit.

without gaining fat. A slow metabolic rate means that you probably burn up food more slowly and gain fat easily. If you exercise regularly your metabolic rate increases permanently and you burn up any excess calories. Many people put on weight when they start exercising regularly as they build up muscle and burn off fat. This is because muscle is heavier than fat – but at least you can do more with it!

SPORT	calories burned per 30 minutes	good for
Badminton	160	legs, arms, waist
Cycling	175-250	legs
Dancing - ballet	125	all-over toning
- disco	150	thighs, waist, arms
Running	250-350	legs
Skipping	300	legs and arms
Swimming - fast	300	all-over toning
- slow	125	all-over toning
Squash	300	arms, legs, waist
Tennis	175	arms, legs, waist
Walking (fast)	125	legs
Weight training	300-400	all-over toning

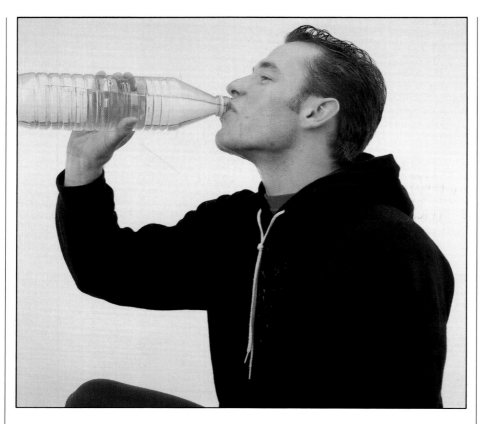

additives, salt and caffeine. If you eat a varied diet with plenty of fresh food then you will absorb the tiny amounts of vitamins and minerals needed to keep your body functioning well.

◄ After exercise you need to replace body fluids lost through sweating.

Drinking plenty of water every day is good for you and it's cheap.

Getting started

Once you have decided to change in these small ways then you can start to build in some regular form of exercise. Choose something that you can really enjoy and which makes you feel good. You need to be able to do it regularly - for 20 to 30 minutes, two or three times a week. Your exercising needs to fit well into your daily routine so that there's no excuse for not keeping it up. Make sure that you can exercise near home so that you don't have to travel too far. Most importantly, choose the kind of exercise that

You are what you eat

What you eat affects your health. A balanced diet is one which has plenty of variety. You need protein, found in foods such as lean meat, nuts, dairy products and pulses. Protein builds new cells and repairs damaged tissue as well as supplying energy. Carbohydrates also provide you with energy. They are found in foods such as bread, pasta, cereals, fruit and root vegetables. Your diet should also include plenty of fibre, found in fruits, vegetables, wholewheat bread, rice, beans and nuts. Fibre keeps your digestive system healthy. It fills you up and speeds up digestion. You need only a small amount of fat in your diet. Animal fats contain cholesterol which can cause fatty deposits in arteries.

Try replacing animal fats with vegetable fats, (called polyunsaturated fats). Other foods to avoid in excess are sugar, food

It's never too late!

It's never too late to get started. A few simple changes in lifestyle - in what you eat and drink, and the amount of exercise you take - can work wonders. Start by asking yourself whether you are as active as you could be in your daily life. For example, do you stand in a bus queue or sit in a traffic jam when you can walk or cycle? Do you use the stairs instead of the lift and do you walk up escalators? Are you the kind of person who always asks someone else to get up and pass you something when you could get it yourself? If you are, how about a change?

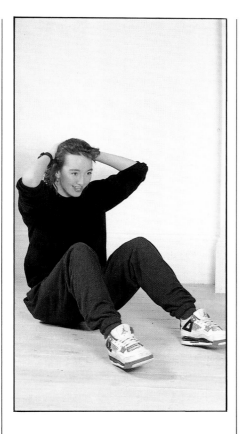

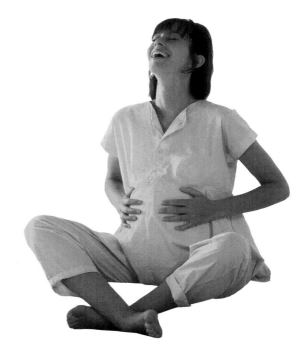

◀ Exercise can be great fun and very good for you. However, it is easy to get carried away and try too much too soon. You could damage your knees or back by doing certain exercises incorrectly. It is important to warm up and keep your knees slightly bent in any exercise that could damage your back.

▲ There is always some kind of exercise you can do at every stage of your life.

▼ An energetic approach to life is the key to a healthy body and mind.

allows you to begin gently and work up gradually, day by day and week by week.

Take care !

Start gradually and always warm up first. Ask your doctor about exercising if you have asthma or bronchitis, back trouble, pains in your joints, diabetes, if you are recovering from an illness or operation or you are worried that exercise might affect any other aspect of your health. Don't do any vigorous exercise for at least an hour after a meal. Don't exercise if you have a cold, temperature or sore throat and start back again gradually when you feel better. Stop exercising if you have pain, dizziness or if you feel unusual tiredness, or at all sick or unwell.

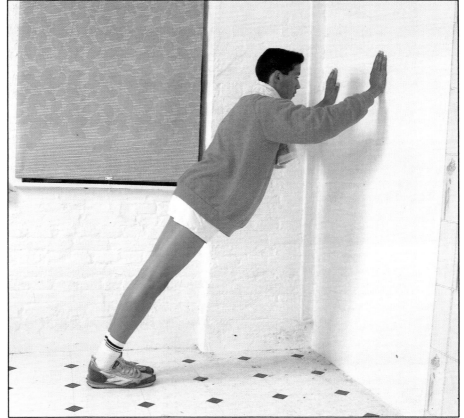

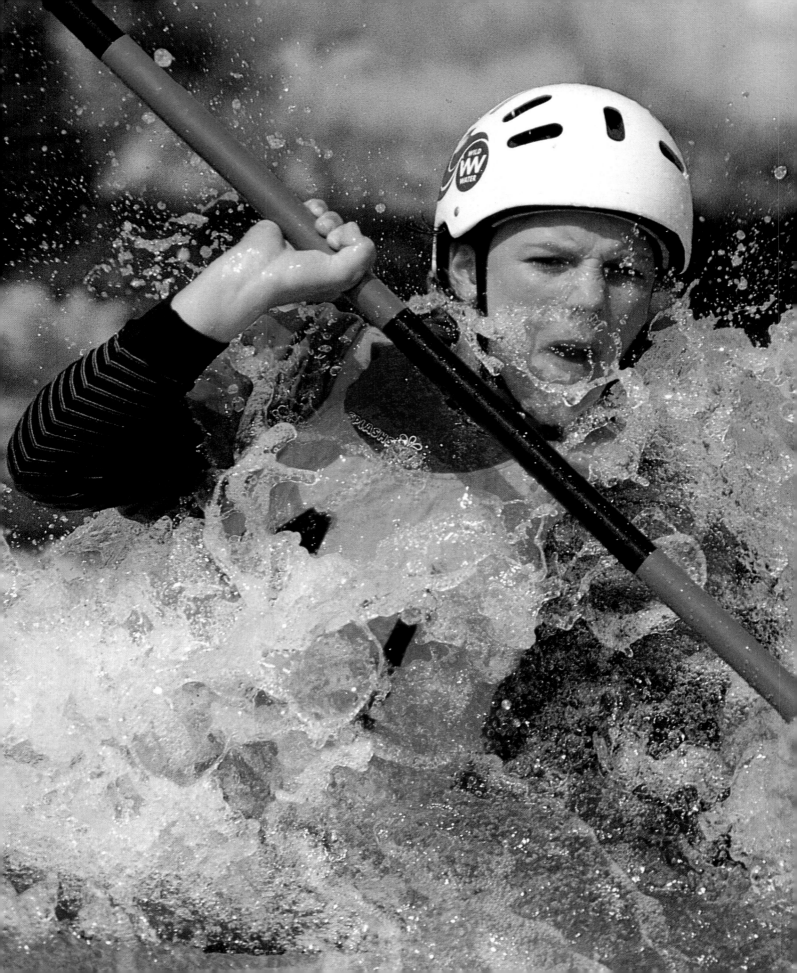

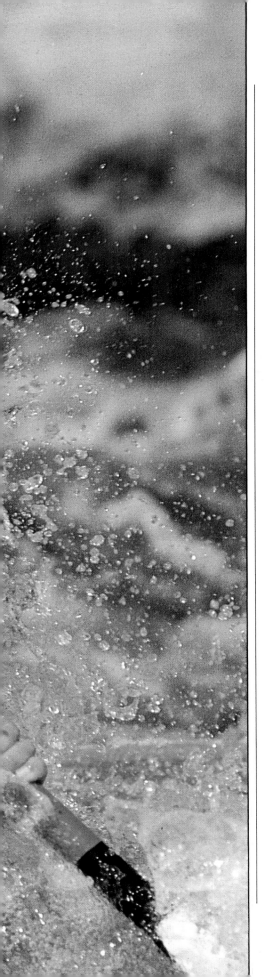

EXERCISING

For stamina, strength and suppleness

Why stamina ?

A good level of stamina gives you more energy, which means you can keep going longer during exercise without tiring. As you exercise, you gradually strengthen your heart and lungs, and other muscles, making them become more efficient. This improves your stamina.

Step it up !

Stamina-developing exercise is called aerobic exercise. Aerobic activities should make you feel fairly breathless. Running up and down stairs or simple repetitive exercise such as stepping up on to a stair and down again both improve stamina. Try improving your stamina by walking more often. Walk briskly and make sure that your shoes are comfortable. More vigorous, continuous exercise such as jogging, skipping, cycling and swimming all increase stamina and strengthen muscles. As your stamina improves you will find yourself

◀ Competitors in this white water canoe race need well developed arm, shoulder and neck muscles to combat the strength of the water.

▶ Steffi Graf needs plenty of stamina to survive three gruelling sets of tennis.

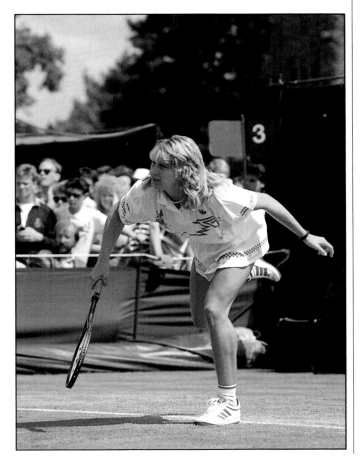

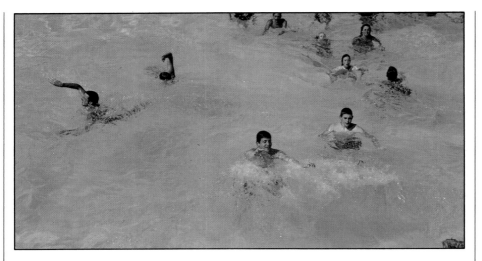

increasing your work load and feeling less breathless. Try measuring your stamina by checking your performance. (See page 21)

Why strength ?

Exercising for strength means toning up the 600 or so muscles in your body. The object is not to have bulging biceps but to keep all your muscles in good shape. Weak muscles in your stomach and back put unnecessary strain on your spine, leading to back pain. Strong stomach muscles mean good posture which avoids back pain as well as flattening out any bulges! Strong arms are necessary for pushing, pulling and lifting actions. Strong leg muscles mean you can catch the bus every time you are late meeting a friend, instead of watching it roar off into the distance while you fight for breath on the pavement.

An easy way to increase strength is to do exercises which use your body weight, such as sit-ups, press-ups and squat jumps.

▲ Swimming is one of the best ways of developing all-round fitness - and it's fun!

▼ Working out in the gym should be done under supervision to avoid injury.

Start by repeating the exercises five or six times, and slowly build up to about 20 repeats when you are really fit.

Exercise machines

These are useful for building up strength and stamina. Try one out at your local sports centre; buying your own can be very expensive. Stationary bikes have the same exercise value as cycling. But cheaper versions don't have adjustable saddles and handlebars. You need to be able to choose how hard to push, so check that the bike has adjust-able resistance on the pedals.

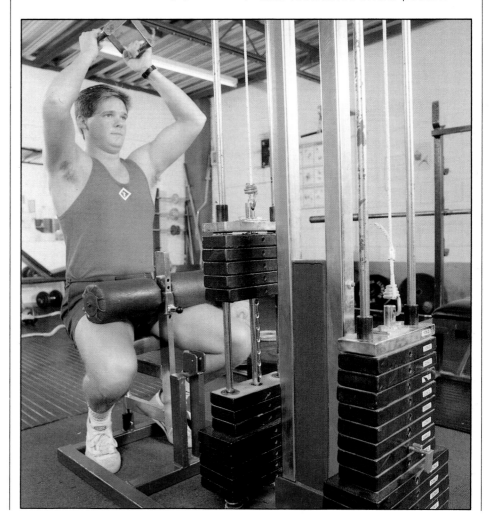

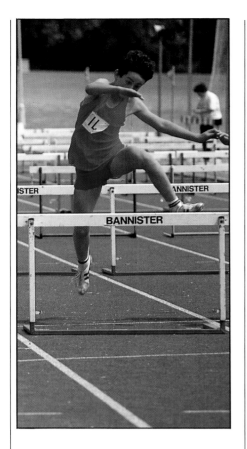

Why suppleness ?

Suppleness is very important in everyday life. Being supple means that you can lift, stretch and bend down smoothly. Stretching exercises help to retain suppleness in old age when joints stiffen up. Exercises to improve suppleness should be included in any fitness programme. This is because suppleness reduces the risk of sporting injuries by improving the mobility of your joints, and increasing agility. If you feel self-conscious about your lack of fitness, you can always do stretching exercises at home. When you feel fitter and more confident, then you can think about joining a club or class.

Gentle stretching exercises should be performed slowly. They are often used for warming up before an exercise session. Activities such as volleyball, skiing, skating, dancing, gymnastics, judo, yoga, tennis and swimming are particularly good at keeping you supple.

◀ Exercising badly is worse than not exercising at all! If you want to get fit, do it properly. Warm up before exercise and cool down afterwards.

▼ Yoga improves suppleness and is a great way to relax. It is a form of exercise which can be done anywhere; even in your own bedroom.

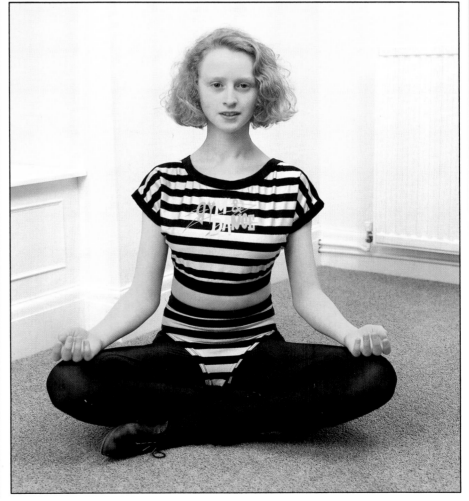

Rowing machines strengthen legs, back and shoulders and are also good for improving stamina.

A carefully designed weight training programme increases strength. But exercising badly is worse than not exercising at all. Serious injury can result from lifting heavy weights without advice from a qualified instructor. The instructor or sports coach will advise you on which machines to use, ensuring that the correct muscle groups are being worked. Never progress to heavier weights until you have mastered the techniques of lifting. Exercising to improve strength does not mean that the activity should be long or painful. You should feel the exercises working but not hurting.

STAYING FIT

Fit for life ?

You are only half-way there if you manage to get fit. Once you are fit you have to make sure that you stay fit - for life! When it becomes natural for you to lead an active life, staying fit is less of a problem. Don't choose just one activity, try out lots of different ones. This means that you are more likely to have a good balance of exercises to improve all three of the elements of fitness - suppleness, strength and stamina.

If you want your body to remain healthy for life then you have to look after yourself by avoiding things that can harm it.

Smoking, stress and a poor diet can lead to heart disease. Habitual excessive drinking and taking non-medical drugs are guaranteed to cause you a number of mental and physical problems. Alcohol is high in calories and heavy drinkers risk being overweight as well as causing damage to their livers.

Sleep, rest and relaxation

Just as important as exercise and healthy eating is the time you give your body to recharge itself through rest and sleep. Your mind and body are active all the time you are awake and need time to rest. Lack of sleep affects your concentration and performance during the day. During sleep hormones are released which stimulate body tissues to grow and repair themselves.

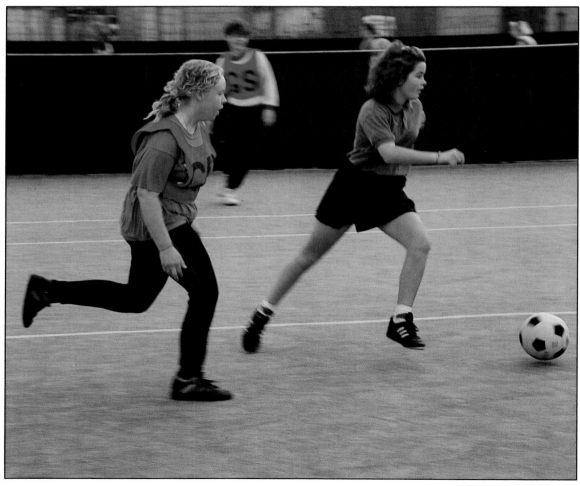

◄ Make sure that you choose an enjoyable activity that's right for you.

▶ Warming up exercises are vital for loosening up before strenuous exercise.

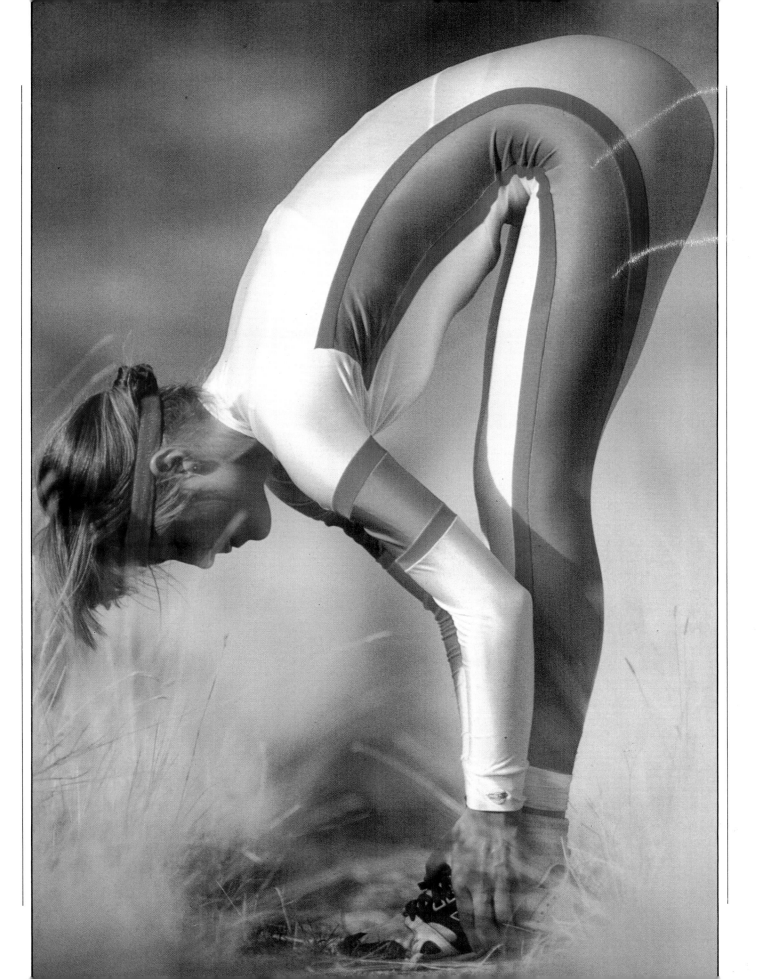

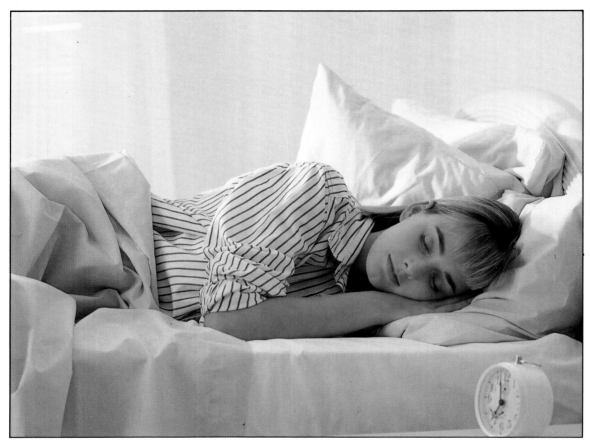

◀ To stay healthy you need to recharge your batteries with plenty of sleep.

▼ Keeping fit and healthy will give you more energy to go out and enjoy yourself.

Teenagers need at least eight hours sleep a night. Younger children need more sleep because they have even more growing to do. After a late night try having an early one the following night to catch up on your sleep.

Mind and body

Your mental health is just as important as your physical health, and the two are closely related. It's important to feel good about yourself. Regular exercise helps with this by making you feel more positive, refreshed and active. Make sure that you don't set yourself targets that are too high, though. Be realistic, and if you fail to reach a target then aim lower

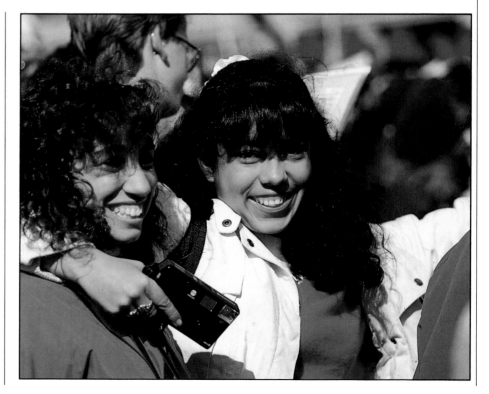

next time. Avoiding stressful situations is part of the art of learning to pace yourself. Learning to relax is very important too. Luckily, feeling more relaxed is just one more of the positive side-effects of exercising.

Test your fitness

After you have started exercising regularly you can test your fitness to see how much you have improved. One clear indication of improved fitness is whether you feel able to exercise for longer, so that at the end of a session you feel that you could easily do some more. Seeing how quickly your pulse rate returns to normal after exercising is another good indicator of fitness. As you become fitter and your heart becomes stronger, your pulse rates at rest and during exercise become lower.

Take your pulse at rest and record the result. Then take it immediately after exercise and see how long it takes to return to the original number of beats per minute. Your pulse should be around 60 beats per minute at rest for a male and around 70 beats for a female. Obviously the heart's capacity to perform declines with age. A fit 20-year-old can let the pulse rise to 170 beats a minute without problems. A fit 50-year old may not feel comfortable with a pulse above 140. Your pulse should return to normal within one or two minutes, depending on the amount of exercise taken.

Fitness test (1): Walk briskly up and down a flight of about fifteen stairs three times. How breathless

▼ This warm-up exercise will help to loosen up your muscles, before you begin more strenuous exercise. If you do not warm up before hand, you risk straining muscles and perhaps doing yourself a serious injury. Keep your knees slightly bent to avoid straining your back.

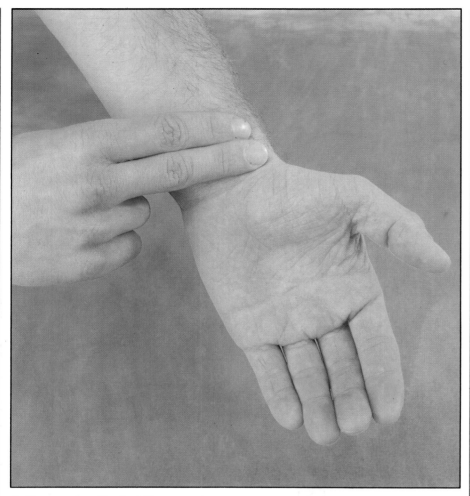

▲ The correct position for taking your pulse.

are you afterwards? So breathless that you cannot speak or just slightly troubled by the test? If you were only a little breathless try the next test:

Fitness test (2): Choose a step about 15 cm high. Step up and down about 24 times a minute for three minutes. Stop for one minute and then measure your pulse rate. Check it against the table below.

male	female	
<72	<80	excellent
72-80	80-90	good
83-100	91-112	average
>100	>112	poor

Warm up and cool down
Before you do any kind of exercise you need to get extra blood flowing to your muscles by doing warm-up exercises. Warming up prepares your body, getting any stiffness out of your joints and muscles before the hard work begins. Warm up by stretching and relaxing the muscles and joints that you are going to use. Warming up before exercising and winding down afterwards avoids risk of injuries. Winding down exercises give your body time to settle down. Remember to put on warm clothes after exercising. At first you may feel rather hot and sweaty. Your body continues to try to get rid of the heat produced when energy is released as you use your muscles. Wrapping up warmly helps prevent what can be a harmful, sharp drop in body temperature.

Warm up

Here is an easy warm-up exercise. Stand up straight with your feet together and go up on to tiptoe while raising your arms from your sides. Push your arms up and stretch. Then gently lower your arms and heels. Repeat the exercise slowly several times.

Tone up

Here are some easy body-shaping exercises that, used regularly, will keep your muscles well toned. Do as many repetitions as you can, building up to around 20 of each.

a. Waist: Stand with your feet wider than your hips, knees slightly bent and your hips tilted forward, bottom tucked in. Keep your hips facing the front and twist round your torso with your arms at shoulder height. (See opposite page.)

b. Legs: Lie flat on your back with your hands on the floor at your sides and your legs up in the air as near to a right angle as you can. Keeping your legs straight, move them apart as far as it feels comfortable without straining. Move them gradually back together again.
(See opposite page.)

c. Stomach and shoulders: Lie on your back with your arms at your sides, knees bent and feet hip-width apart. Breathe in, and then as you breathe out, lift your head and shoulders off the ground, making sure that you keep your back flat by tilting your hips upwards. Gently lower your head and shoulders.

Cool down

After exercising allow your body to cool down gently by slowing down your movements until you are still and relaxed. This helps to avoid stiffness later. Finally rest by lying on the floor for a few minutes in a comfortable position.

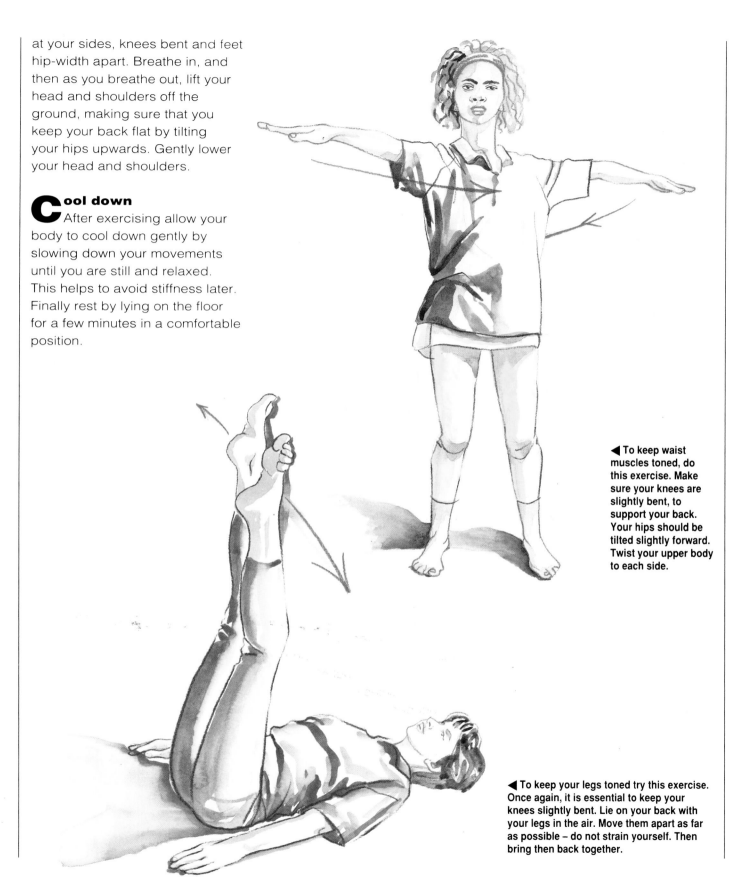

◀ To keep waist muscles toned, do this exercise. Make sure your knees are slightly bent, to support your back. Your hips should be tilted slightly forward. Twist your upper body to each side.

◀ To keep your legs toned try this exercise. Once again, it is essential to keep your knees slightly bent. Lie on your back with your legs in the air. Move them apart as far as possible – do not strain yourself. Then bring then back together.

GO FOR IT!

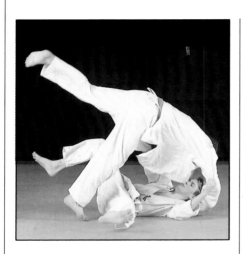

Choosing the right kind of exercise for you depends on whether you like being in contact with a lot of people, whether you like solitary outdoor pursuits, or whether you prefer taking exercise in small groups or with one friend. Getting into shape does not have to mean puffing your way through punishing work-outs or joining expensive clubs and classes. There are hundreds of activities on offer. Here are just a few.

Home sweet home

There is no place like home for starting off a new fitness campaign. There are a wide variety of fitness tapes, books and videos available. Check out your local library or the health and fitness section of your nearest record, video or book shop. Another simple way of staying fit is skipping. A few minutes a day as part of your daily routine is easy, cheap and especially good for your heart.

Stepping out

Taking exercise outside in the fresh air is not just good for you – it is free! Walking is one of the easiest ways to keep fit. It is a great way to explore the countryside and is an activity that can be enjoyed by all ages. Make sure that you take a long, brisk walk, exerting yourself enough to raise your pulse rate slightly. Jogging is perfect for increasing your stamina. Your local park is a good place to run and is better than jogging alongside the traffic in the city centre. It is safer, and can be more fun, to jog with a friend. It is better to jog on softer ground than on a hard road too. The impact of your feet on the road surface can damage your joints and spine.

Pedal power

Cycling is cheap, fast, healthy and, like walking, kind to the environment! It is particularly good for strengthening the muscles in your legs and back. Bikes are cheap to maintain, and often cheap to buy. You might find a second-hand one advertised in your local paper. There are lots of cycling clubs you can join which offer short trips and cycling holidays.

Make sure you cycle safely by maintaining your bike carefully and following the highway code. Always wear a cycling helmet to protect your head, and a reflective band so that you can be seen easily, especially if you cycle at night.

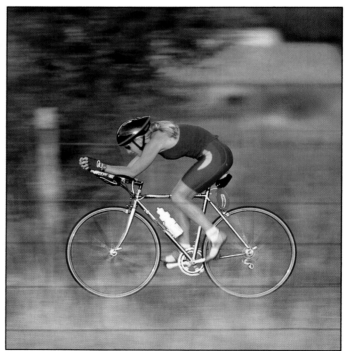

▲ TOP LEFT
When you choose a sport, bear in mind that some require expensive training and specialized equipment and clothing.

◄ **You can spend a great deal of money on fashionable sports gear. However, the basics are well fitting shoes and comfortable clothing that doesn't catch in equipment.**

► **Exercise can be a very sociable activity. Marathon running has become popular for all age groups.**

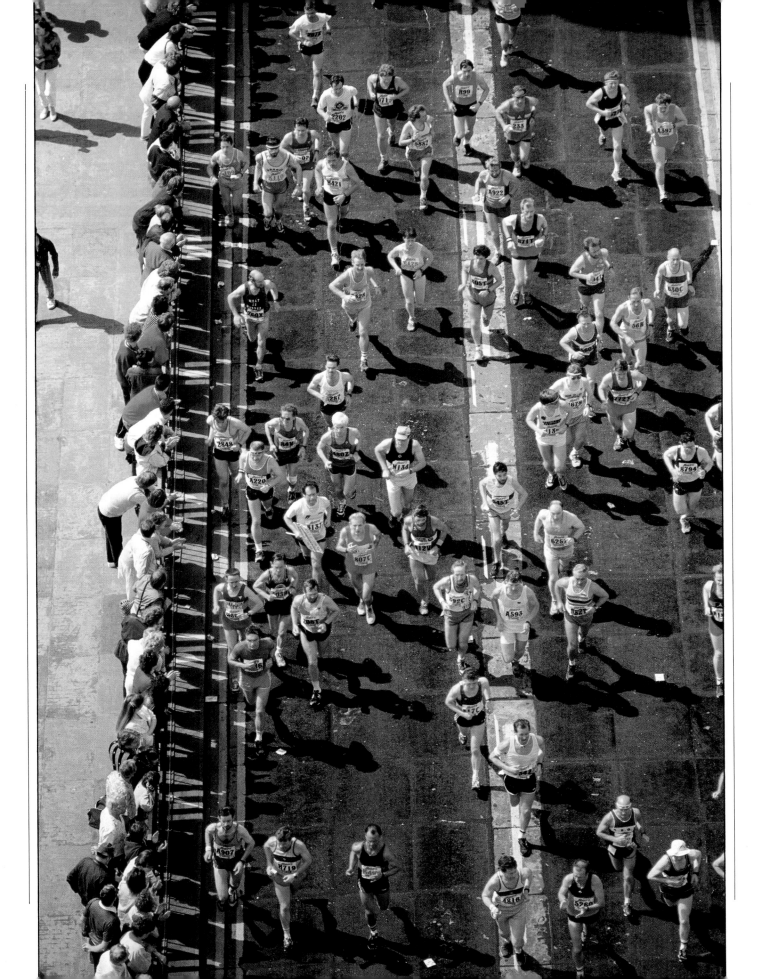

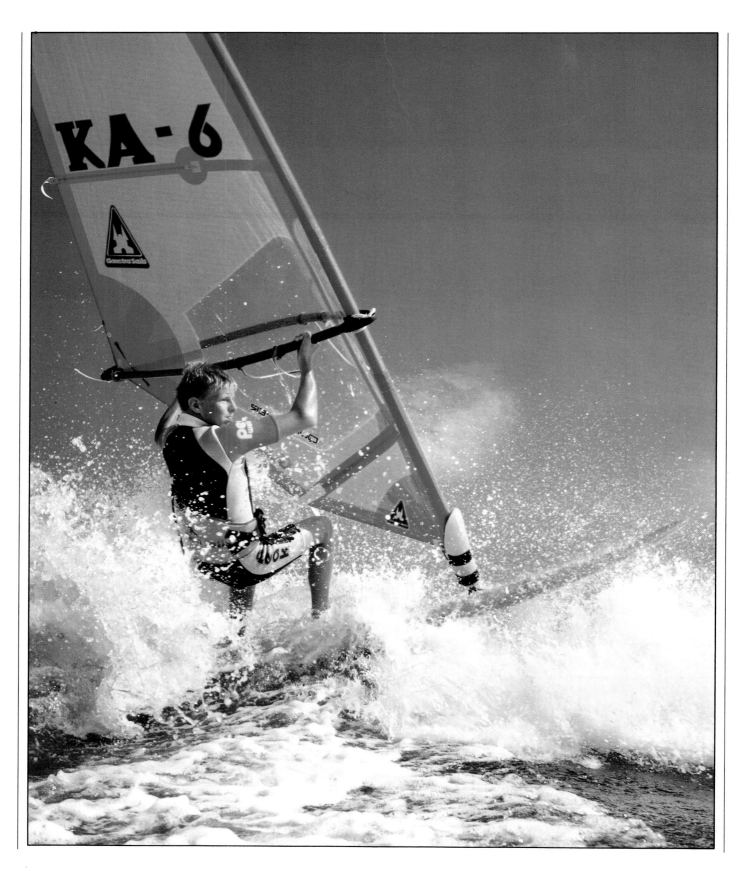

Make a splash

For an activity that combines the three areas of fitness - strength, suppleness and stamina - you can't beat swimming. Swimming is a very popular activity, ideal for people of all ages and an excellent way to get fit and have a good time. Don't be put off if you can't swim well. Most pools offer classes for all ages. You might like to try aquarobics, an alternative form of aerobics in water. It uses the resistance of the water to strengthen and tone up your muscles.

In the gym

Perhaps working out in the gym is more your style. Try joining a local sports centre and use its gym. Sports centres usually have

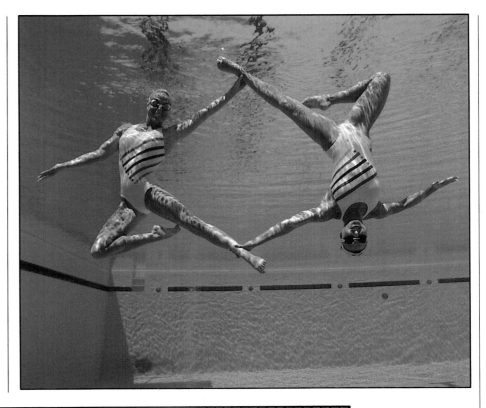

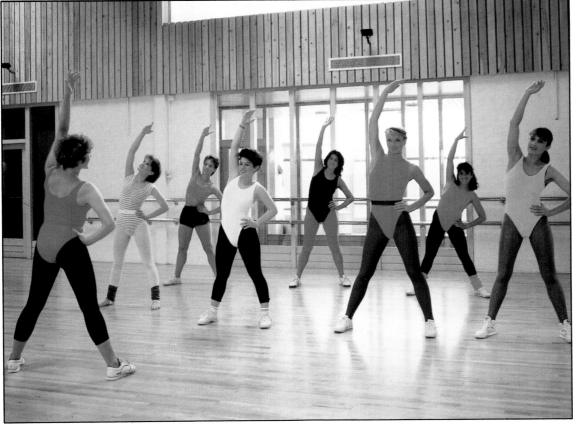

▲ Healthy hearts and lungs are essential to synchronized swimmers who need to control their breathing in order to perform.

◀ If you decide to take up aerobics, try to find a group which has a gym with a spring floor. This is far better for your joints.

◀ OPPOSITE PAGE Exercising in fresh air and the challenge of pitting yourself against the elements can be exhilarating.

exercise machines, weight training and circuit training equipment. Often you are asked to do a simple fitness test so that an expert can prepare an exercise plan to suit your needs; it is important not to over-do it. A wide variety of fitness classes for all ages are offered at sports centres. Aerobics classes combine jogging and jumping for stamina with stretching and strengthening exercises for an all-round work-out. Moving to music is great fun and a good way of meeting people. Dancing classes are another excellent way of improving your fitness.

▼ Basic sports gear is a good investment, if you decide to take up a sport.

▶ The dedication and single mindedness needed to reach the top of any sporting activity is more than most people are willing to give.

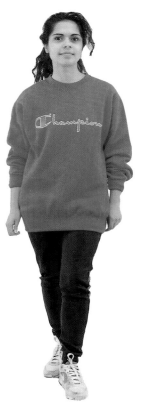

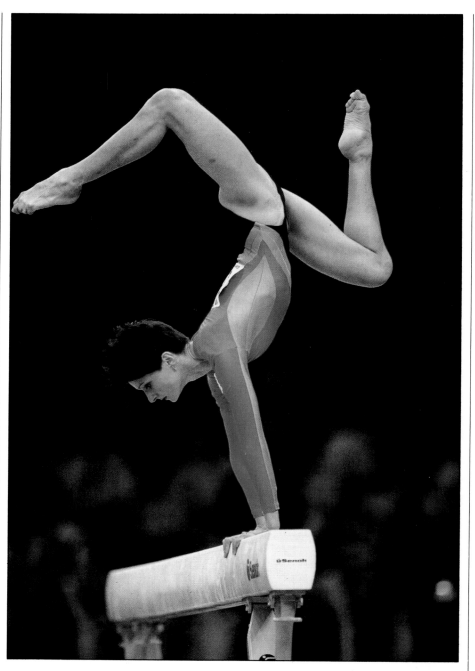

Sports wear

Wearing suitable clothing that keeps you warm while exercising is important. If you are cold it means that your body is using up valuable energy to warm you up. This makes you feel unnecessarily tired. Being cold also cuts down the supply of blood to your muscles and can result in injury. Layers of clothes are a good idea, enabling you to peel off items as you warm up.

If you have decided to choose an active lifestyle, treat yourself to something new such as a track-suit or leotard to start you off. Remember loose clothes are more comfortable. Track suits are useful for warming up in and putting on after exercising. Shorts and T-shirts allow freedom of movement. Avoid clothes made from uncomfortable materials which do not absorb sweat. Several fabrics have been specially developed for sports wear, such as lycra which is both stretchy and comfortable. It allows freedom of movement. A good pair of trainers is a sound investment. Trainers should offer strong support to your heels and arches. Make sure that they are properly fitted by an expert at a sport shop and *not* in a fashion store.

There's no stopping you now

There is no limit to the ways in which you can get fit. Tennis, rounders, cricket, badminton,

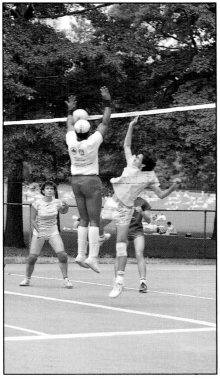

◀ Your health shows in every aspect of your behaviour and appearance. Go for the glow!

▲ The fitter you become, the more energy you will have to enjoy yourself.

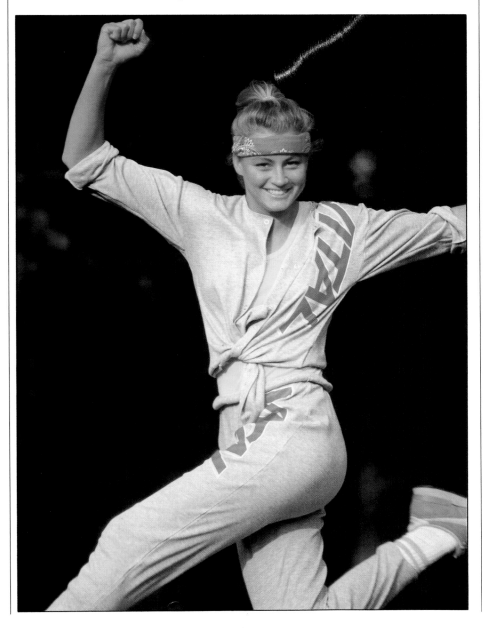

football, it's up to you! Team games are a very good way of meeting people, although some of them depend on the seasons or the weather and are not always a reliable part of a fitness campaign. Many alternative leisure activities are good for fitness. Getting into shape does not always mean fierce exertion. You may prefer activities that require a more meditative approach like yoga or meditation.

Whatever you choose to do, make sure that you enjoy it. This means that you will want to carry on. The most important thing to remember is that you can't store fitness - to keep fit you have to keep active. Good luck!

GLOSSARY

Aerobic exercise Exercise that strengthens your heart and lungs.

Arteries Arteries are blood vessels which carry oxygenated blood from the heart around the body.

Caffeine A stimulant found in coffee and tea.

Calories Units of measurement of the energy in food.

Cholesterol A substance in the body which can block the arteries and increase the risk of heart disease.

Hormones Chemical substances produced by the body which control its functions.

Posture The position of your limbs and body; the way you hold yourself.

Pulse The pumping action of the heart. The pulse rate is the rate at which your heart beats.

Stamina Staying power.

Suppleness The ability to bend, move or twist easily.

Torso The trunk of the human body, not including the head or limbs.

BOOKS TO READ

You and Your Fitness and Health, by Kate Fraser and Judy Tatchell
(Usborne Publishing Limited, 1986)
Exercise and Fitness by Brian R Ward (Franklin Watts, 1988)
Everygirl's Lifeguide by Miriam Stoppard
(Dorling Kindersley Limited, 1987)
Health and Fitness in Focus by Hilary Tunnicliffe (Franklin Watts, 1991)
Choosing Health by Alan Collinson (Cloverleaf, an imprint of Evans
Brothers Limited, 1991)
People and Energy by Jan Burgess (Macmillan Education Ltd, 1987)
Diet and Health by Ida Weekes (Wayland, 1991)

FURTHER INFORMATION

You can find out more about the sporting facilities in your area from your sports centre or swimming pool, your local library, the Leisure or Recreation Department of your Local Authority, your social club, your local newspaper or your Local Health Education Unit. Their telephone numbers can be found in the phone book. The Health Education Unit number is listed under your District Health Authority.

For more general information about specific sports ring the Sports Council Regional Office that serves your county:

Greater London and South East
Sports Council
Tel: (081) 778 8600

Sports Council for Wales
Tel: (0222) 397571

Sports Council for Northern
Ireland
Tel: (0232) 661222

Scottish Sports Council
Tel: (031) 225 8411

For help and advice on giving up smoking, contact:
Action on Smoking and Health
(ASH)
5-11 Mortimer Street,
London W1N 7RH

Other useful addresses:
Look After Yourself Project Centre
Christ Church College,
Canterbury,
Kent CT1 1QU
Tel: (0227) 455564
They will tell you the number of your regional office.

Health Education Authority
78 New Oxford Street,
London WC1A 1AH

British Heart Foundation
14 Fitzhardinge Street,
London W1H 4DH

The British Sports Association for
the Disabled (BSAD)
34 Osnaburgh Street,
London NW1 3ND
Tel: (071) 383 7277

Cyclist Touring Club
Cotterell House,
69 Meadrow,
Godalming,
Surrey GU7 3HS
Tel: (0483) 417217

INDEX

Picture Acknowledgements

Action Plus 8; All Sport 6,7,10 (bottom); Cephas 4; Chapel Studios 12,16 (top and bottom),17 (bottom),20 (bottom),22,28 (bottom); Eye Ubiquitous 18 (left); Life file 13 (top, left), 17 (top, left); Paul Skjold 7,11; Tony Stone *cover*,9,10 (top),13 (top),14, 15, 20 (top),24 (bottom),25,26,27 (top and bottom),28 (top),29 (bottom); Wayland Picture Library 5,13 (bottom),24 (top); Zefa 19,29 (top). Artwork by Debbie Hinks.

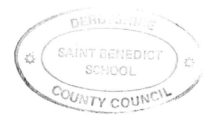